POCKET ATLAS OF NORMAL ULTRASOUND ANATOMY

Second Edition

Pocket Atlas of Normal Ultrasound Anatomy

Second Edition

Matthew D. Rifkin, MD

Professor of Urology
Professor and Vice Chairman of Radiology
Chief of Diagnostic Radiology
School of Medicine
State University of New York at Stony Brook
Stony Brook, New York

Mani Montazemi, RDMS

Clinical Instructor
Jefferson Ultrasound Research and Education Institute
Thomas Jefferson University Hospital
Philadelphia, Pennsylvania

Robert Villani, MD

State University of New York at Stony Brook
Stony Brook, New York

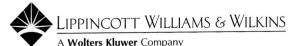

LIPPINCOTT WILLIAMS & WILKINS

A **Wolters Kluwer** Company

Philadelphia • Baltimore • New York • London
Buenos Aires • Hong Kong • Sydney • Tokyo

Acquisitions Editor: Joyce-Rachel John
Developmental Editor: Ellen DiFrancesco
Printer: Sheridan Press

© 2001 by LIPPINCOTT WILLIAMS & WILKINS
530 Walnut Street
Philadelphia, PA 19106 USA
LWW.com

Library of Congress Cataloging-in-Publication Data

Rifkin, Matthew D.
  Pocket atlas of normal ultrasound anatomy/Matthew D. Rifkin, Mani Montazemi, Robert Villani.—2nd ed.
    p.; cm.
  ISBN 13: 978-0-7817-3029-5
  ISBN 10: 0-7817-3029-5

  1. Human anatomy—Atlases. 2. Ultrasonic imaging—Atlases. I. Montazemi, Mani. II. Villani, Robert, MD. III. Title.
  [DNLM: 1. Abdomen—anatomy & histology—Atlases. 2. Abdomen—anatomy & histology—Handbooks. 3. Genitalia, Male—anatomy & histology—Atlases. 4. Genitalia, Male—anatomy & histology—Handbooks. 5. Neck—anatomy & histology—Atlases. 6. Neck—anatomy & histology—Handbooks. 7. Pelvis—anatomy & histology—Atlases. 8. Pelvis—anatomy & histology—Handbooks. 9. Ultrasonography—Atlases. 10. Ultrasonography—Handbooks. WI 17 R564p 2000]
  QM25 .R545 2000
  616.07′543—dc21   00-064566

10 9 8 7 6 5 4 3 2

Preface

There have been great improvements in ultrasound equipment since the publication of the first edition. While normal anatomy has not changed, the development of new ultrasound transducers has allowed imaging access to the body in different orientations than previously possible. Therefore, this atlas has in many instances, provided a number of images of the body in similar planes, in order to account for angulation of the transducer, body habitus, and variation in normal anatomy. As in the previous edition, this handbook focuses on the neck, abdomen, pelvis, and also includes images of the external male genitalia.

Contents

Neck

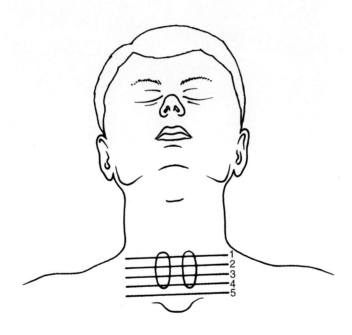

Transverse Planes T1–T5

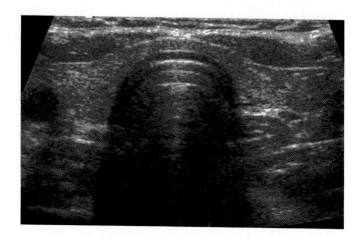

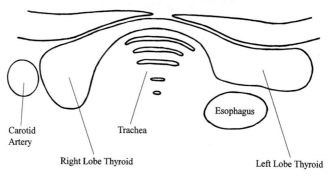

Carotid
Artery

Trachea

Right Lobe Thyroid

Esophagus

Left Lobe Thyroid

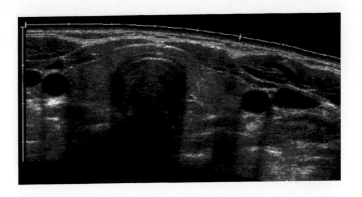

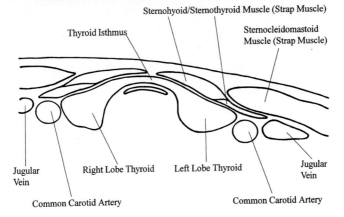

Sternohyoid/Sternothyroid Muscle (Strap Muscle)

Sternocleidomastoid
Muscle (Strap Muscle)

Thyroid Isthmus

Jugular
Vein

Right Lobe Thyroid

Left Lobe Thyroid

Jugular
Vein

Common Carotid Artery

Common Carotid Artery

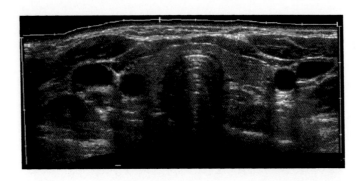

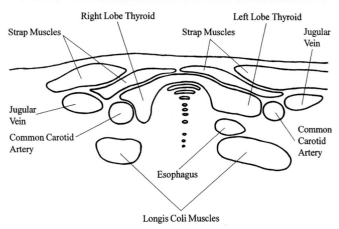

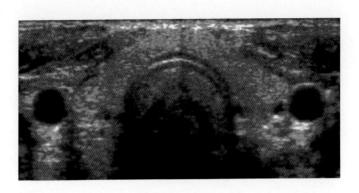

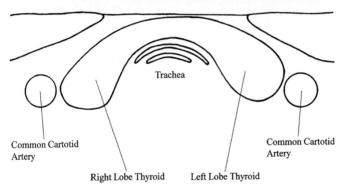

Trachea

Common Cartotid
Artery

Common Cartotid
Artery

Right Lobe Thyroid   Left Lobe Thyroid

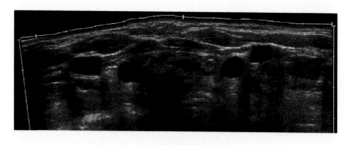

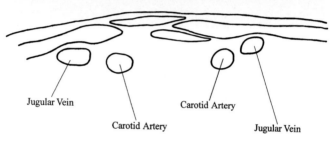

Jugular Vein

Carotid Artery

Carotid Artery

Jugular Vein

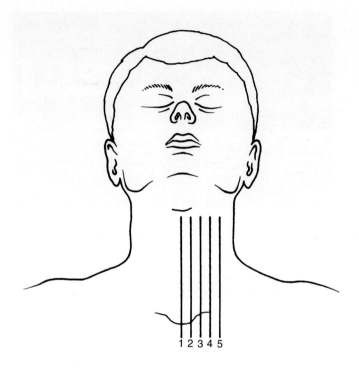

1 2 3 4 5

Sagittal Planes S1–S5

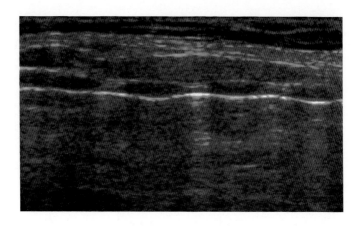

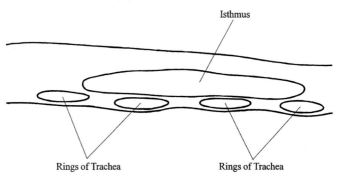

Isthmus

Rings of Trachea　　　　　Rings of Trachea

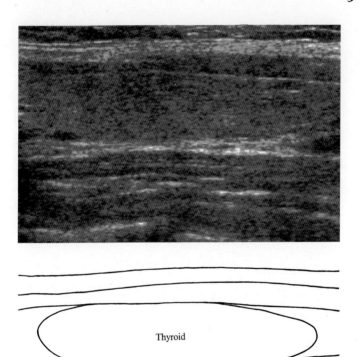

Thyroid

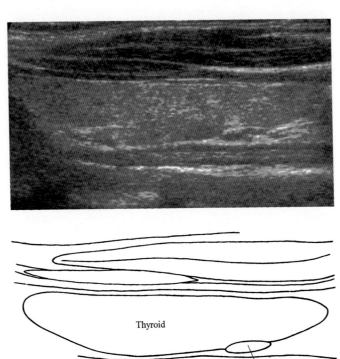

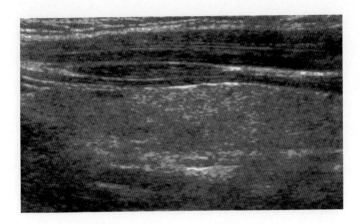

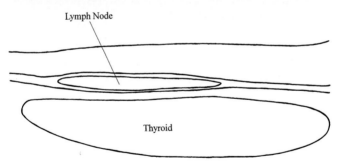

Lymph Node

Thyroid

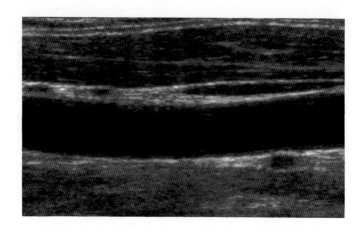

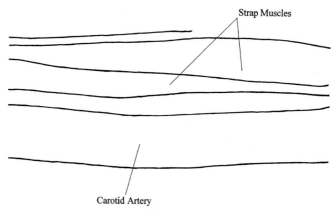

Strap Muscles

Carotid Artery

Abdomen

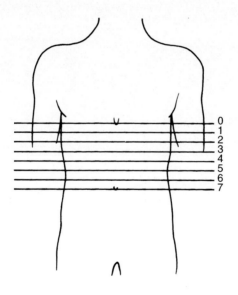

0
1
2
3
4
5
6
7

Transverse Planes T1–T7

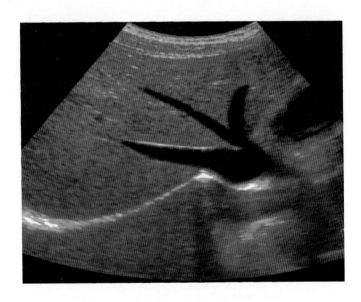

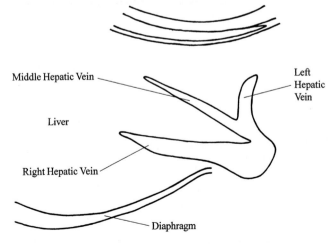

Middle Hepatic Vein

Left Hepatic Vein

Liver

Right Hepatic Vein

Diaphragm

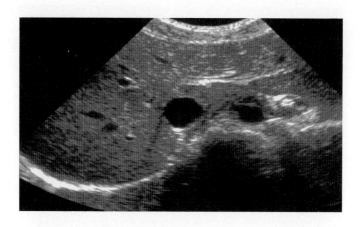

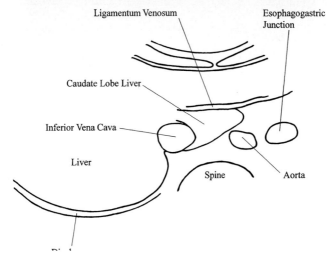

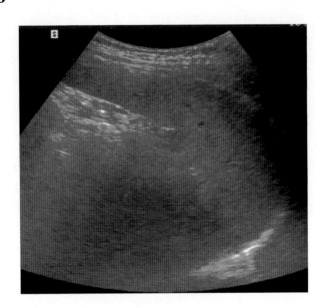

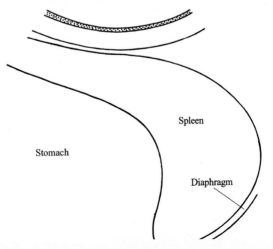

Spleen

Stomach

Diaphragm

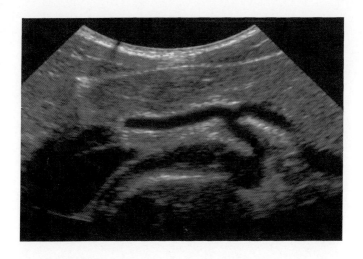

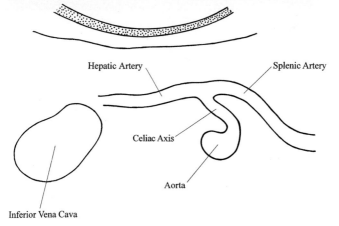

Hepatic Artery

Splenic Artery

Celiac Axis

Aorta

Inferior Vena Cava

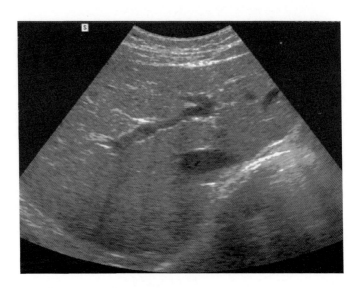

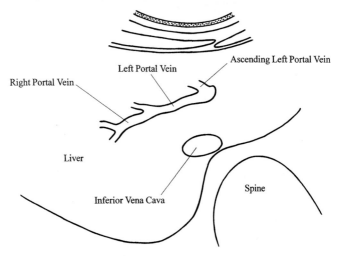

Ascending Left Portal Vein

Left Portal Vein

Right Portal Vein

Liver

Inferior Vena Cava

Spine

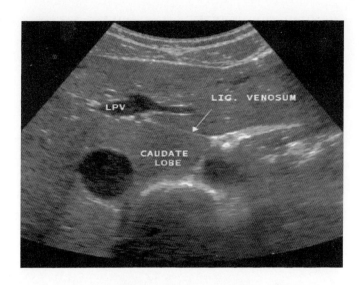

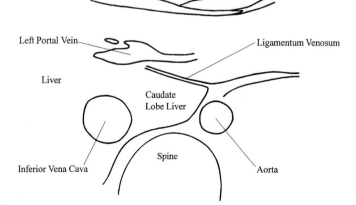

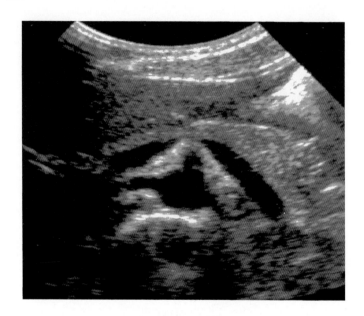

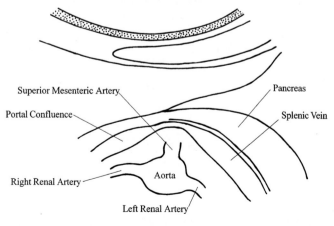

Superior Mesenteric Artery

Portal Confluence

Right Renal Artery

Aorta

Left Renal Artery

Pancreas

Splenic Vein

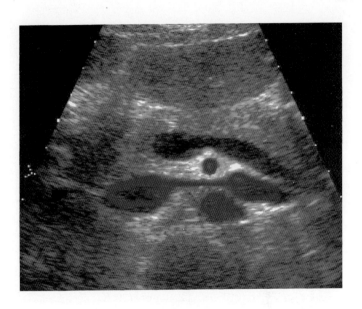

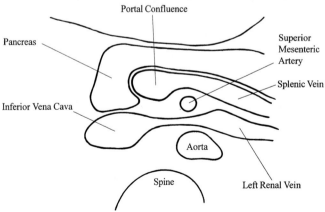

Portal Confluence

Pancreas

Superior
Mesenteric
Artery

Splenic Vein

Inferior Vena Cava

Aorta

Left Renal Vein

Spine

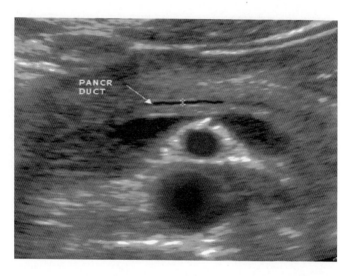

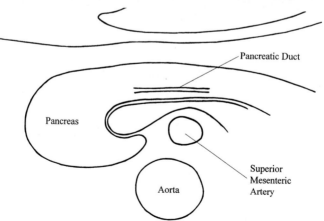

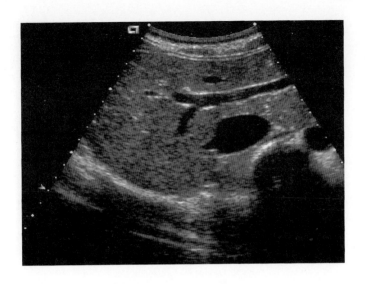

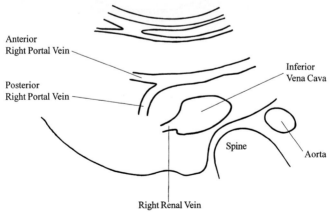

Anterior
Right Portal Vein

Posterior
Right Portal Vein

Inferior
Vena Cava

Aorta

Spine

Right Renal Vein

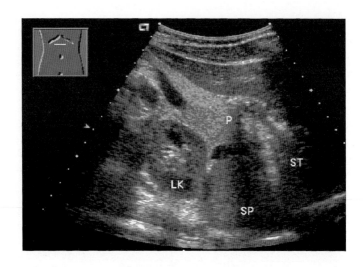

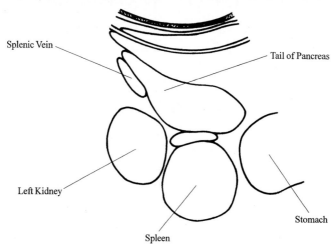

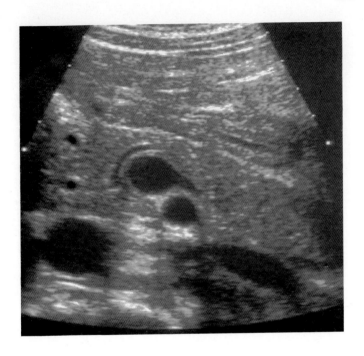

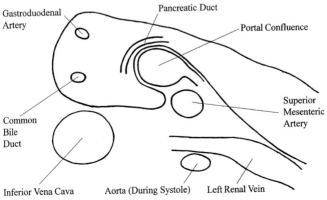

Gastroduodenal Artery

Pancreatic Duct

Portal Confluence

Common Bile Duct

Superior Mesenteric Artery

Inferior Vena Cava

Aorta (During Systole)

Left Renal Vein

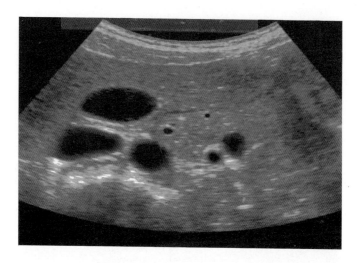

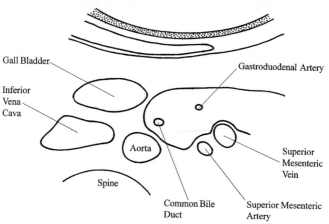

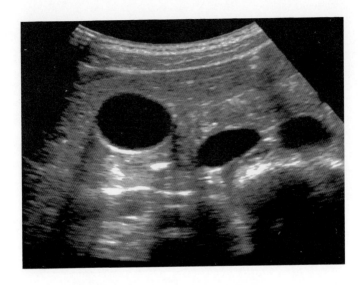

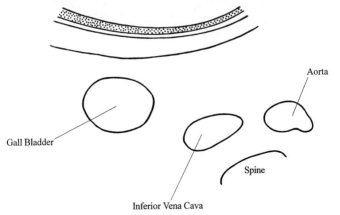

Aorta

Gall Bladder

Inferior Vena Cava

Spine

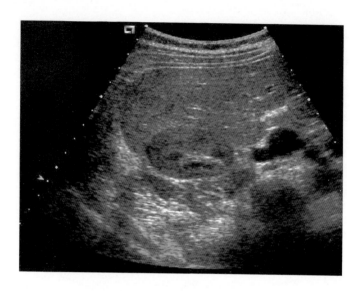

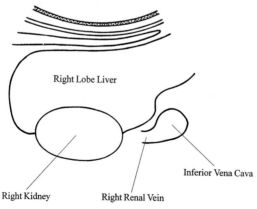

Right Lobe Liver

Inferior Vena Cava

Right Kidney

Right Renal Vein

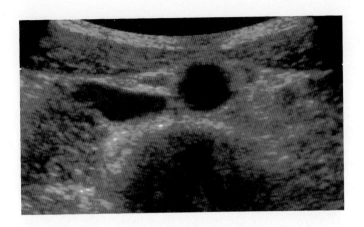

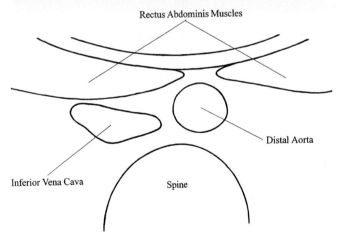

Rectus Abdominis Muscles

Distal Aorta

Inferior Vena Cava

Spine

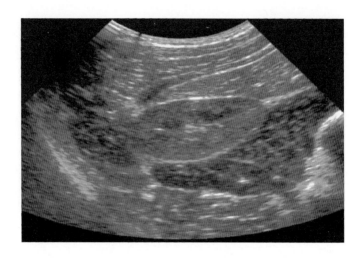

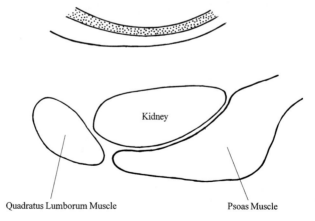

Kidney

Quadratus Lumborum Muscle

Psoas Muscle

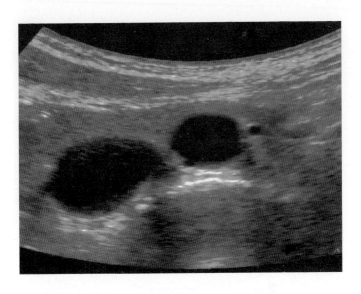

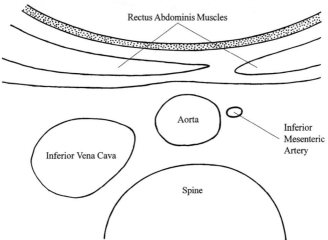

Rectus Abdominis Muscles

Aorta

Inferior Mesenteric Artery

Inferior Vena Cava

Spine

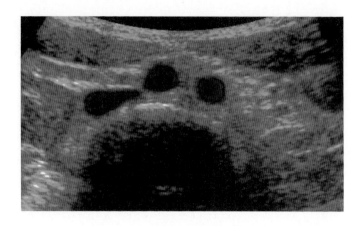

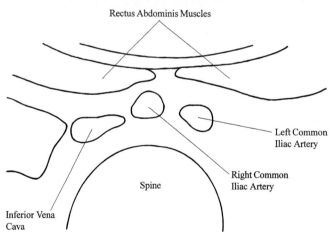

Rectus Abdominis Muscles

Left Common
Iliac Artery

Right Common
Iliac Artery

Spine

Inferior Vena
Cava

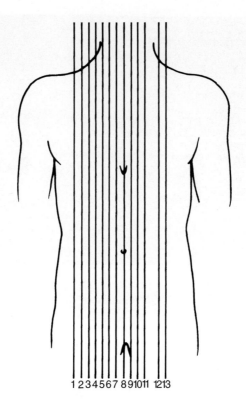

1 2 3 4 5 6 7 8 9 10 11 12 13

Sagittal Planes S1–S13

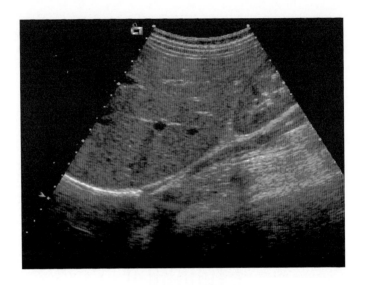

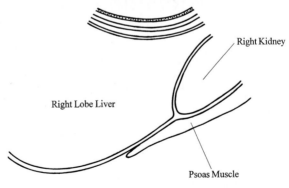

Right Kidney

Right Lobe Liver

Psoas Muscle

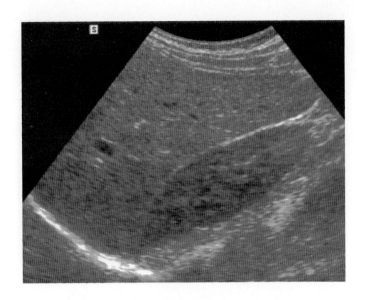

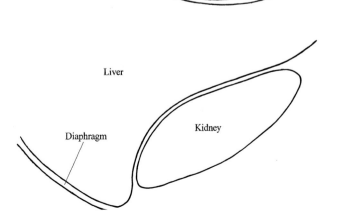

Liver

Diaphragm

Kidney

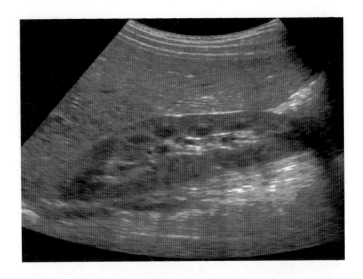

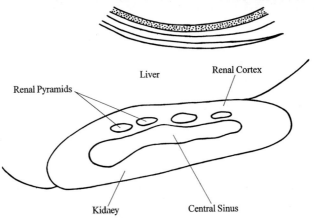

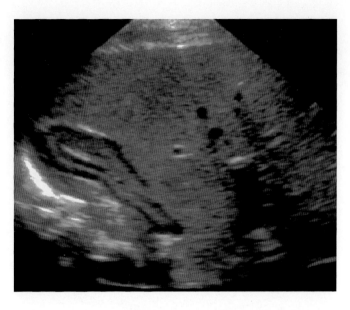

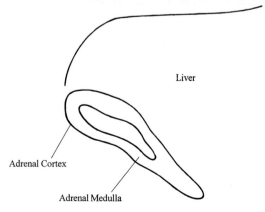

Liver

Adrenal Cortex

Adrenal Medulla

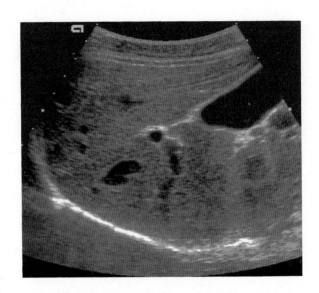

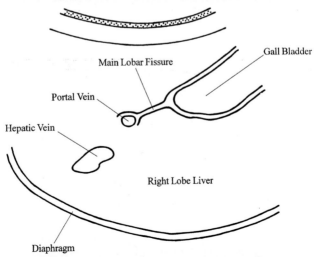

Main Lobar Fissure

Gall Bladder

Portal Vein

Hepatic Vein

Right Lobe Liver

Diaphragm

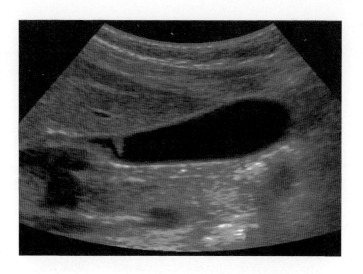

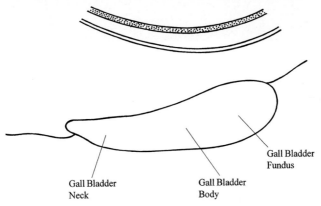

Gall Bladder
Neck

Gall Bladder
Body

Gall Bladder
Fundus

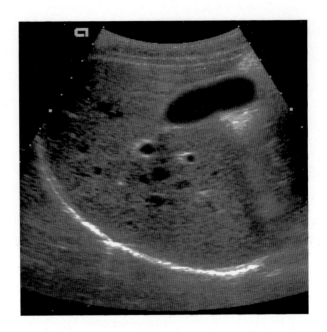

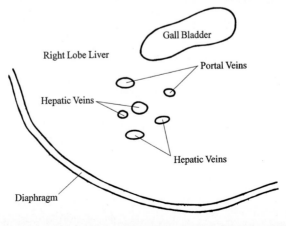

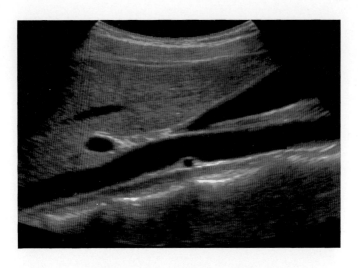

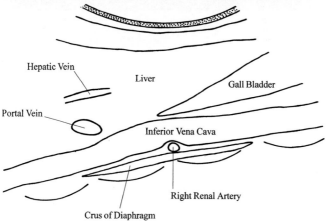

Hepatic Vein

Liver

Gall Bladder

Portal Vein

Inferior Vena Cava

Right Renal Artery

Crus of Diaphragm

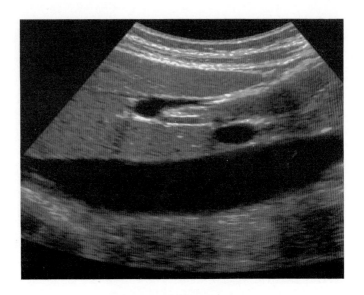

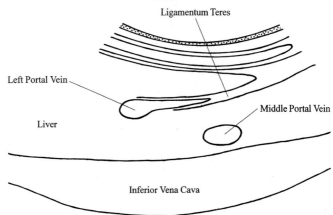

Ligamentum Teres

Left Portal Vein

Liver

Middle Portal Vein

Inferior Vena Cava

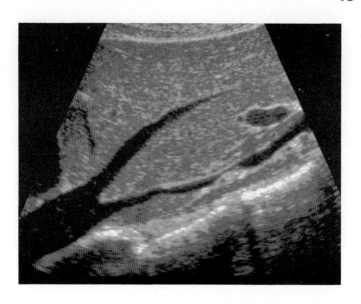

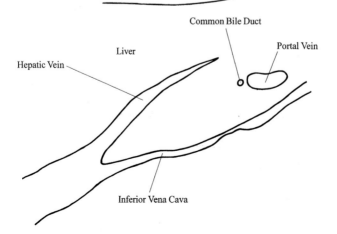

Common Bile Duct

Portal Vein

Liver

Hepatic Vein

Inferior Vena Cava

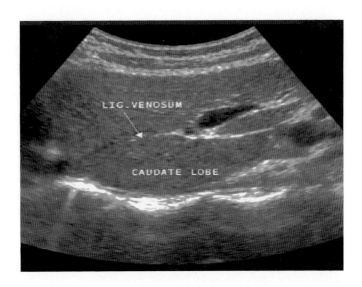

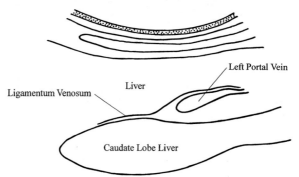

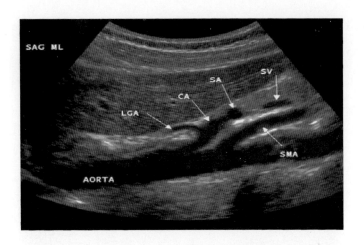

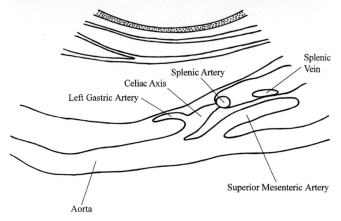

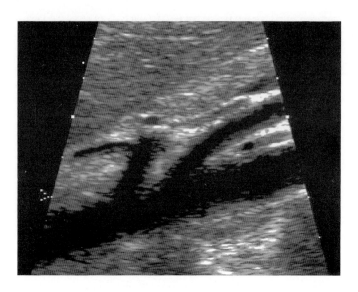

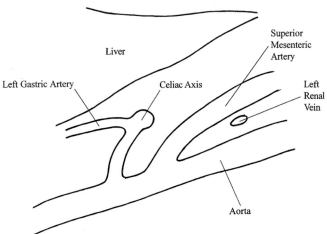

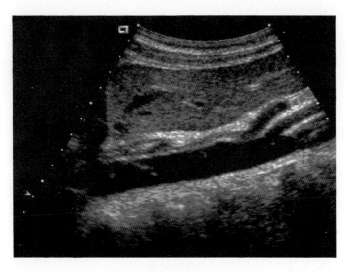

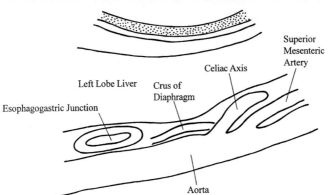

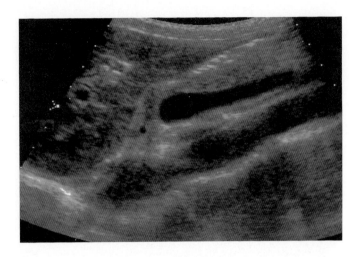

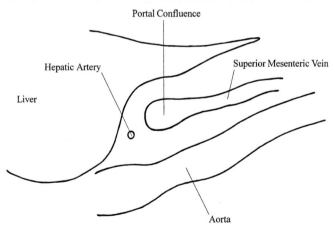

Portal Confluence

Hepatic Artery

Superior Mesenteric Vein

Liver

Aorta

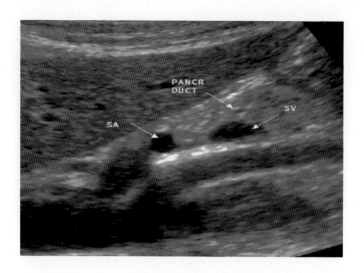

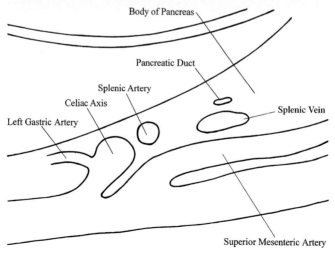

Body of Pancreas

Pancreatic Duct

Splenic Artery

Celiac Axis

Splenic Vein

Left Gastric Artery

Superior Mesenteric Artery

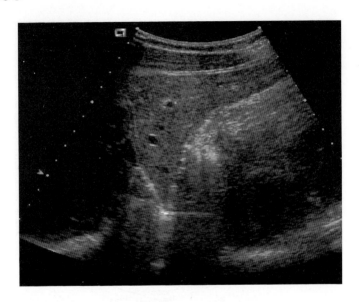

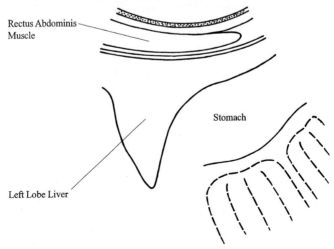

Rectus Abdominis
Muscle

Stomach

Left Lobe Liver

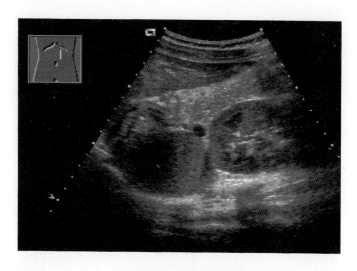

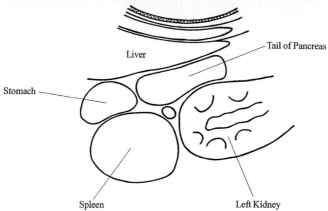

Liver

Tail of Pancreas

Stomach

Spleen

Left Kidney

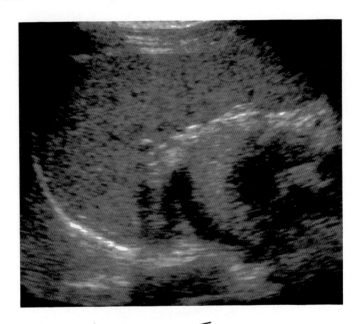

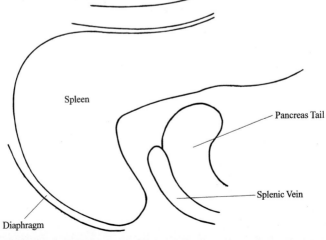

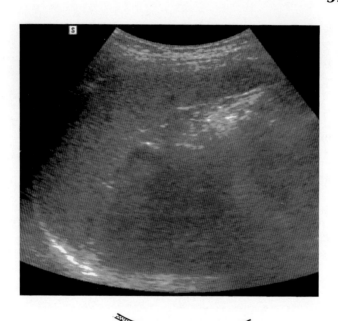

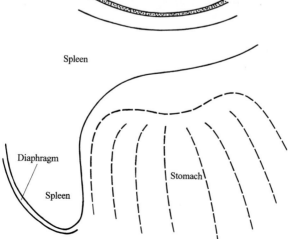

Spleen

Diaphragm

Spleen

Stomach

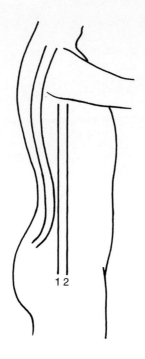

Coronal Planes C1–C2

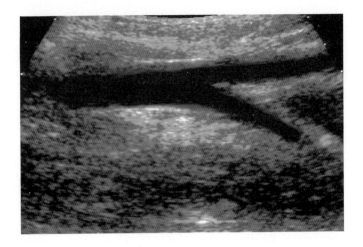

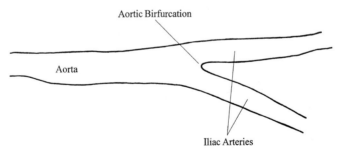

Aortic Birfurcation

Aorta

Iliac Arteries

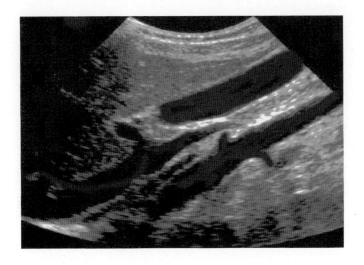

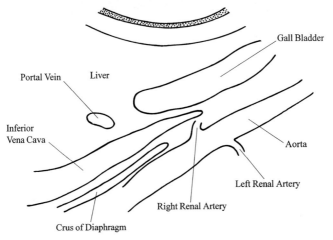

Gall Bladder

Portal Vein   Liver

Inferior
Vena Cava

Aorta

Left Renal Artery

Right Renal Artery

Crus of Diaphragm

Female Pelvis

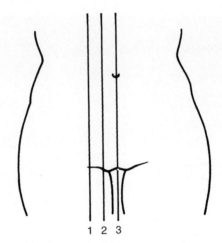

Sagittal Planes S1–S3

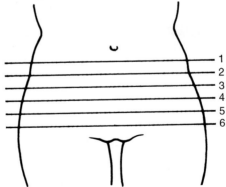

Transverse Planes T1–T6

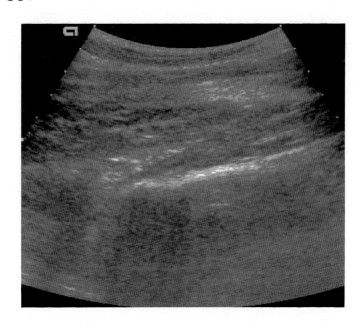

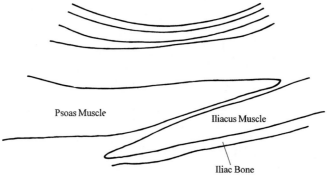

Psoas Muscle

Iliacus Muscle

Iliac Bone

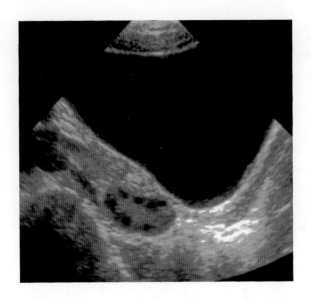

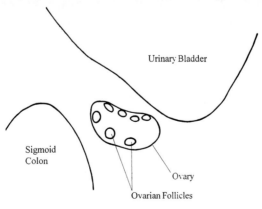

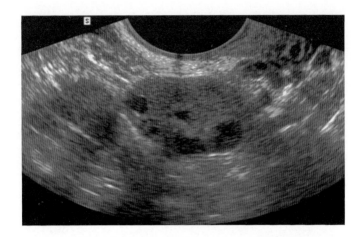

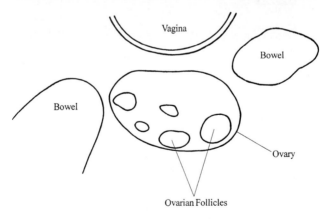

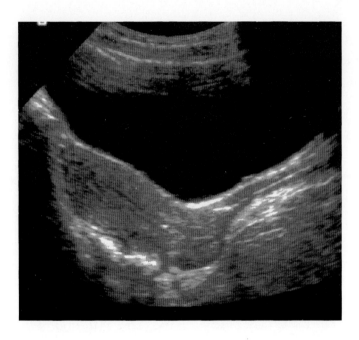

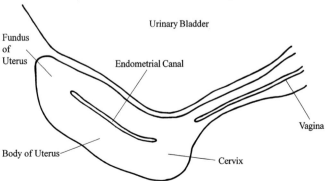

Urinary Bladder

Fundus
of
Uterus

Endometrial Canal

Vagina

Body of Uterus

Cervix

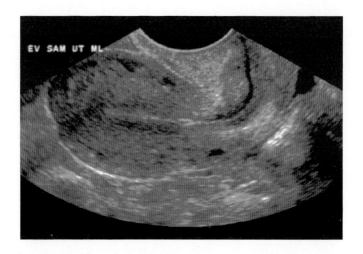

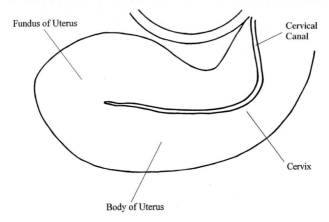

Fundus of Uterus

Cervical Canal

Cervix

Body of Uterus

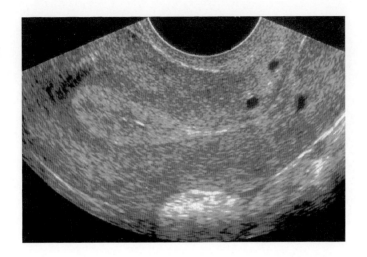

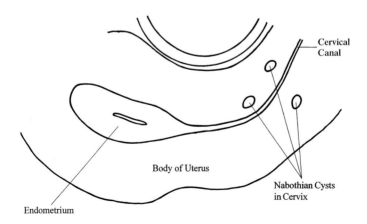

Cervical Canal

Endometrium

Body of Uterus

Nabothian Cysts in Cervix

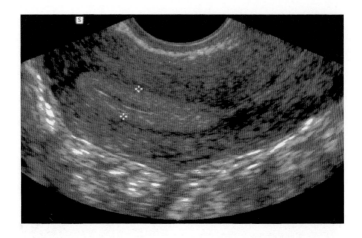

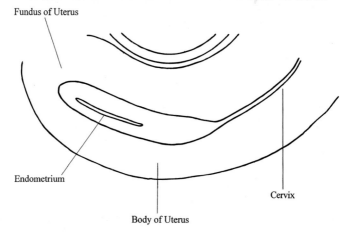

Fundus of Uterus

Endometrium

Body of Uterus

Cervix

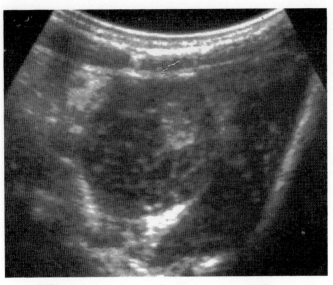

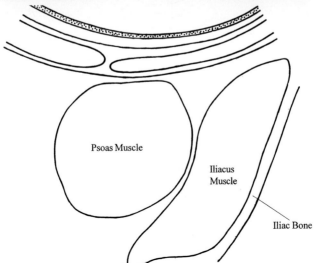

Psoas Muscle

Iliacus
Muscle

Iliac Bone

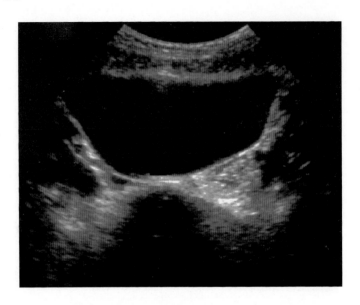

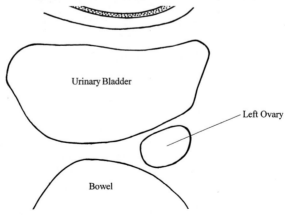

Urinary Bladder

Left Ovary

Bowel

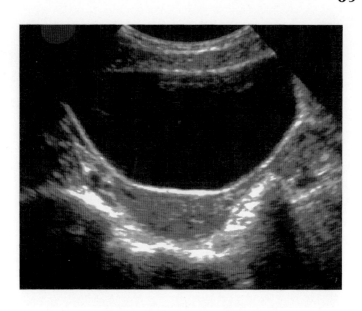

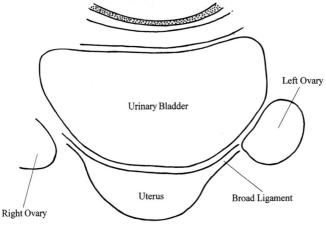

Left Ovary

Urinary Bladder

Uterus

Broad Ligament

Right Ovary

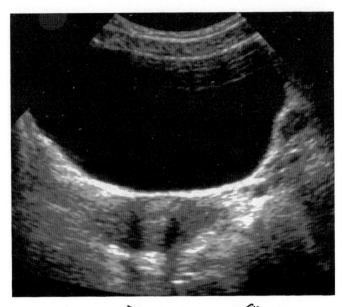

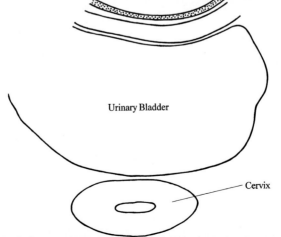

Urinary Bladder

Cervix

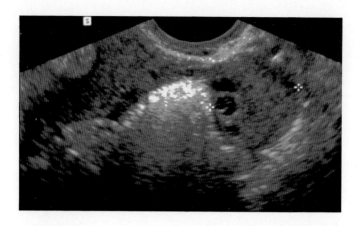

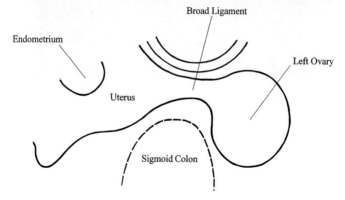

Broad Ligament

Endometrium

Left Ovary

Uterus

Sigmoid Colon

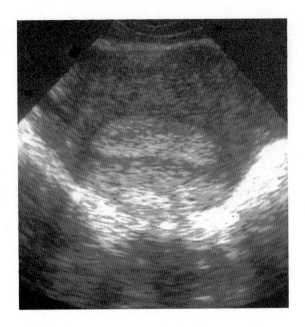

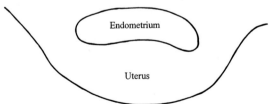

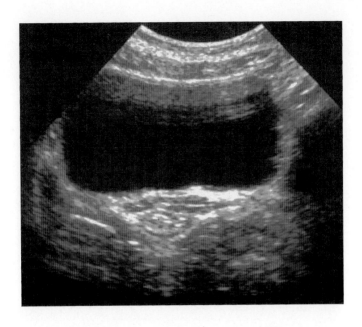

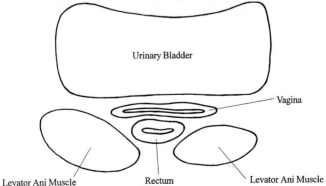

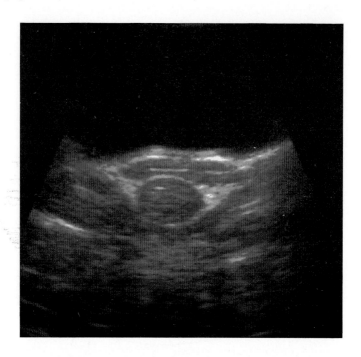

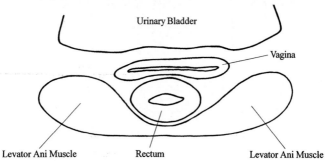

Urinary Bladder

Vagina

Levator Ani Muscle

Rectum

Levator Ani Muscle

External Male Genitalia

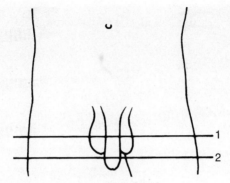

Transverse Planes T1–T2

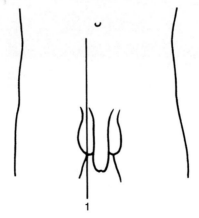

Sagittal S1

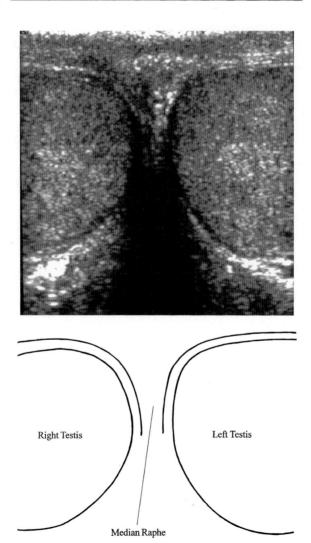

Right Testis

Left Testis

Median Raphe

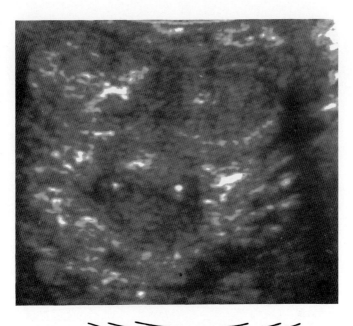

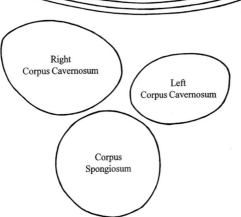

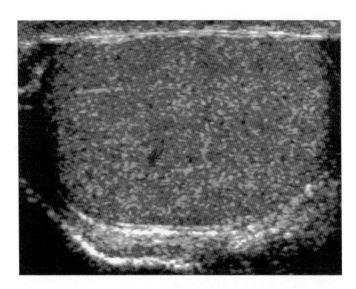

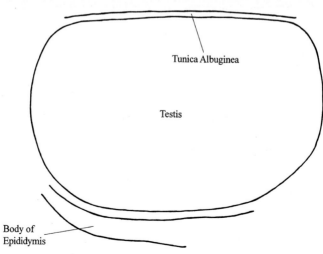

Tunica Albuginea

Testis

Body of
Epididymis

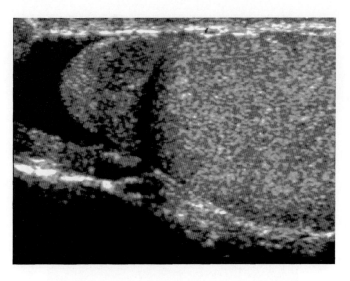

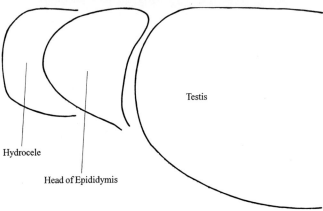

Hydrocele

Head of Epididymis

Testis

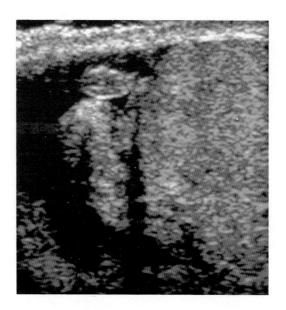

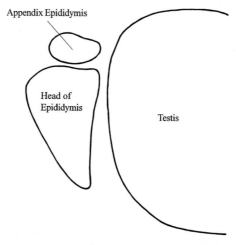

Appendix Epididymis

Head of
Epididymis

Testis